UNLOCKING PELVIC POWER

A Comprehensive Guide to
Effective Pelvic Floor Exercises for
Women and Men - Strengthen,
Restore, and Thrive

Dr. Raymond F. Bernard

TABLE OF CONTENTS

CHAPTER 1

pelvic floor exercises

Welcome to the journey of discovering and strengthening your pelvic floor! In this first chapter, we'll delve into the intriguing world of the pelvic floor - an essential part of your body that often goes unnoticed until problems arise. We'll explore its anatomy, understand its function, and lay the foundation for the empowering knowledge you'll gain throughout this book.

Anatomy of the Pelvic Floor: A Closer Look at What Lies Beneath Picture the bottom of your pelvis, the area between your hip bones. This region is home to a network of muscles, tissues, and ligaments collectively known as the pelvic floor. Think of it as a supportive hammock that cradles and holds your pelvic organs - the bladder, uterus (for women), and rectum. While this area might seem insignificant, the pelvic floor's role is anything but. It supports your core, helps control bodily functions, and contributes to your overall stability.

The Function of the Pelvic Floor: A Balancing Act for Health Imagine standing up, sneezing, or laughing. Did you know that your pelvic floor plays a crucial role in preventing unwanted leaks? Yes, it's your body's natural guardian against urinary incontinence. But that's not all - it also helps regulate bowel movements, contributes to sexual function, and even aids in supporting your abdominal organs. Just like any other muscle group, the pelvic floor needs exercise to stay strong and functional.

The Significance of a Strong and Healthy Pelvic Floor

Imagine a building with a solid foundation. The pelvic floor serves as your body's foundation, and if it's weak or compromised, a range of issues can arise. For instance, pregnancy and childbirth can put stress on the pelvic floor, potentially leading to issues like pelvic organ prolapse. Aging, obesity, and certain medical conditions can also affect pelvic floor health. However, fear not - the power to strengthen and maintain your pelvic floor lies in your hands.

Setting the Tone for the Book: Goals and Structure As we embark on this journey together, keep in mind the goals of this book. We aim to provide you with the knowledge, tools, and exercises to achieve a strong and healthy pelvic floor. We'll tackle various exercises, nutrition tips, and lifestyle changes that can make a significant impact on your pelvic floor health. By the time you finish this book, you'll have a comprehensive understanding of your pelvic floor, its significance, and the steps you can take to nurture it.

In Summary This opening chapter has laid the groundwork for your exploration into the world of pelvic floor health. You now know that the pelvic floor is a complex system of muscles and tissues that play a vital role in maintaining bodily functions, stability, and overall well-being. The following chapters will delve deeper into the benefits of pelvic floor exercises, techniques for strengthening these muscles, and how to integrate healthy habits into your lifestyle. Remember, this journey is about empowerment - by the end of this book, you'll possess the knowledge and tools to take control of your pelvic floor health and live a more confident, active life. So, let's dive into the next chapters and continue our exploration of the incredible pelvic floor!

CHAPTER 2

Getting to Know Your Pelvic Floor

Welcome to Chapter 2, where we're going to take a deeper dive into understanding your pelvic floor. It's like getting to know a new friend; the more you understand it, the better you can care for it. In this chapter, we'll explore how you can assess the state of your pelvic floor, common issues that can arise, and how these issues can affect both men and women.

Self-Assessment: Taking Stock of Your Pelvic Floor

Just as a doctor checks your pulse, it's crucial to get a sense of your pelvic floor's health. There are various ways to do this:

1. **Physical Examination:** You can start with a basic self-examination. Lie down and relax your muscles. Then, insert a clean, lubricated finger into your vagina (for women) or rectum (for men) and contract your pelvic floor muscles. You should feel a gentle tightening around

your finger. If this doesn't happen, it may indicate a weakened pelvic floor.

2. **Observation:** Pay attention to any signs of pelvic floor issues. Do you experience urinary leaks when you sneeze or laugh? Do you have difficulty controlling your bowel movements? These could be indicators that your pelvic floor needs attention.

3. **Consult a Specialist:** If you have concerns or are experiencing symptoms, it's always wise to consult a healthcare provider or pelvic

health specialist. They can perform more thorough assessments and provide personalized guidance.

Common Pelvic Floor Problems Understanding potential issues is the first step in addressing them. Here are some common problems associated with the pelvic floor:

1. **Urinary Incontinence:** This is the unintentional leakage of urine. Stress incontinence occurs during activities like sneezing or laughing, while urge

incontinence is a sudden, strong need to urinate.

2. **Fecal Incontinence:** Similar to urinary incontinence, this involves the unintentional passage of stool.

3. **Pelvic Organ Prolapse:** This occurs when pelvic organs, such as the bladder or uterus, sag or drop into the vaginal canal. It can cause discomfort and affect your quality of life.

4. **Pelvic Pain:** Chronic pelvic pain can result from various causes, including muscle

tension, inflammation, or nerve issues.

5. **Sexual Dysfunction:** A weakened pelvic floor can lead to sexual problems, including difficulty achieving or maintaining an erection or orgasm.

6. **Pelvic Floor Muscle Spasms:** These spasms can cause discomfort, pain, and difficulty with urination or bowel movements.

Gender and the Pelvic Floor

While both men and women have a pelvic floor, they serve slightly different functions and face distinct challenges:

For Women:

- The pelvic floor supports the uterus, which can be affected by pregnancy and childbirth.
- Hormonal changes during menopause can weaken the pelvic floor.
- Pregnancy and childbirth can increase the risk of urinary incontinence and pelvic organ prolapse.

For Men:

- The pelvic floor supports the bladder and rectum.

- Conditions like prostate surgery or an enlarged prostate can impact pelvic floor function.
- Aging can lead to weakening of the pelvic floor muscles in men as well.

It's important to recognize that pelvic floor health matters for everyone, regardless of gender. Both men and women can benefit from exercises and lifestyle changes to maintain or improve their pelvic floor function.

In Summary Chapter 2 has provided an introduction to understanding your pelvic floor.

We've learned how to perform a basic self-assessment, explored common pelvic floor issues, and highlighted that both men and women can be affected. The key takeaway is that knowing your pelvic floor and recognizing potential problems is the first step towards achieving a strong and healthy pelvic floor. In the upcoming chapters, we'll delve deeper into specific exercises and strategies to address these issues and empower you to take control of your pelvic floor health. So, keep reading and get ready to unlock the secrets to a stronger, healthier you!

CHAPTER 3

Benefits of Pelvic Floor Exercises

Welcome to Chapter 3, where we'll explore the numerous benefits of pelvic floor exercises. These exercises aren't just about preventing problems; they can significantly enhance your overall well-being. In this chapter, we'll dive into the advantages of strengthening your pelvic floor muscles, from improved bladder and bowel control to better sexual health and support during pregnancy and postpartum.

Improved Bladder and Bowel Control One of the most significant benefits of pelvic floor exercises is the improvement in bladder and bowel control. For many, this alone is motivation enough to start a pelvic floor workout routine.

- **Urinary Incontinence:** Pelvic floor exercises can help reduce or even eliminate urinary incontinence. Stress incontinence, which causes leaks during activities like sneezing or laughing, often responds well to targeted pelvic floor strengthening. It can be especially beneficial for women who've experienced childbirth, as pregnancy and delivery can weaken these muscles.

- **Overactive Bladder:** An overactive bladder, characterized by frequent and urgent urination, can also benefit from pelvic floor exercises. Strengthening these muscles can help you regain control over your bladder, reducing the urgency and frequency of trips to the restroom.

- **Fecal Incontinence:** Pelvic floor exercises can also aid in the management of fecal incontinence, which involves the unintentional passage of stool. By strengthening the muscles responsible for controlling bowel movements, you can gain better control and confidence.

Enhanced Sexual Health Your pelvic floor muscles play a vital role in sexual function and enjoyment for both men and women.

- **Women:** A strong pelvic floor can improve vaginal tone and sensation, leading to enhanced sexual pleasure. Additionally, these exercises can help with vaginal tightness, which can be particularly beneficial for postmenopausal women.

- **Men:** Pelvic floor exercises can contribute to better erections and greater control over ejaculation. For men dealing with erectile dysfunction, pelvic floor workouts can be a valuable part of a holistic treatment plan.

Support During Pregnancy and Postpartum Pregnancy and childbirth place unique demands on the pelvic floor. Strengthening these muscles can provide critical support during this transformative time.

- **Pregnancy:** Pelvic floor exercises can help support the growing weight of the baby and the uterus. This can reduce the risk of pelvic organ prolapse and urinary incontinence during pregnancy.

- **Labor and Delivery:** Strong pelvic floor muscles can assist in labor and delivery. Women with well-conditioned pelvic floors may experience smoother deliveries and faster recovery times.

- **Postpartum Recovery:** After childbirth, the pelvic floor often requires rehabilitation. Pelvic floor exercises can aid in the healing process, helping women regain control over their bladder and pelvic organs.

Prevention and Management of Pelvic Organ Prolapse

Pelvic organ prolapse occurs when pelvic organs, such as the bladder, uterus, or rectum, sag or descend into the vaginal canal. Pelvic floor exercises can help prevent and manage this condition.

- **Prevention:** Strengthening the pelvic floor muscles can provide vital support to prevent pelvic organ prolapse, especially in women who've had multiple pregnancies or experienced difficult childbirth.

- **Management:** For those already dealing with pelvic organ prolapse, targeted exercises can help manage the condition, alleviate discomfort, and improve quality of life.

In Summary Chapter 3 has illuminated the incredible benefits of pelvic floor exercises. These exercises aren't just about preventing problems; they're about enhancing your overall well-being. By improving bladder and bowel control, enhancing sexual health, and offering support during pregnancy and postpartum, pelvic floor exercises empower you to lead a more comfortable, confident, and fulfilling life. As we progress through this book, we'll delve deeper into the practical aspects of pelvic floor exercises, helping you harness these advantages for yourself. So, let's continue our journey towards a stronger, healthier pelvic floor!

CHAPTER 4

Preparing to Exercise

Welcome to Chapter 4, where we'll lay the foundation for your pelvic floor exercise journey. Just like any fitness program, it's essential to start with the right mindset, equipment, and a comfortable environment. In this chapter, we'll guide you on setting realistic goals, creating an exercise-friendly space, and identifying the necessary equipment and attire to embark on your pelvic floor exercise routine.

Setting Realistic Goals Before you dive into pelvic floor exercises, it's crucial to establish clear and achievable goals. Realistic goals provide direction, motivation, and a sense of accomplishment as you progress in your journey. Here's how to set them:

- **Identify Your Objectives:** Start by identifying what you hope to achieve through pelvic floor exercises. Is it better bladder control? Enhanced sexual function? Or preventing pelvic organ prolapse? Your objectives will shape your exercise routine.

- **Make Them Specific:** Instead of a vague goal like "I want a stronger pelvic floor," make it specific. For instance, "I want to reduce urinary leakage when I laugh or sneeze."

- **Set a Timeline:** Having a timeline creates a sense of urgency and helps you track progress. For example, "I want to see a noticeable improvement in bladder control within three months."

- **Break It Down:** Divide your goals into smaller, manageable steps. This makes your journey less daunting and more achievable.

Creating a Comfortable Exercise Space The environment in which you perform your pelvic floor exercises can significantly impact your success and comfort. Here are some tips for creating a space that promotes consistency and motivation:

- **Privacy:** Choose a private space where you feel comfortable and secure.

Pelvic floor exercises can involve intimate movements, so having a space free from distractions or prying eyes is essential.

- **Lighting:** Ensure the room is well-lit. Good lighting is not only practical but also psychologically uplifting.

- **Comfortable Flooring:** Opt for a comfortable and non-slip surface. Yoga mats or padded exercise mats work well to cushion your movements.

- **Temperature Control:** Maintain a comfortable temperature. You don't want to be too hot or too cold during your exercise routine.

- **Music or Relaxing Sounds:** Some people find that background music or soothing sounds like ocean waves enhance their exercise experience. Consider incorporating these into your exercise space.

Necessary Equipment and Attire Pelvic floor exercises are simple and can often be done without any equipment. However, a few items can enhance your comfort and effectiveness:

- **Exercise Wear:** Wear comfortable clothing that allows for freedom of movement. You don't need anything special; just ensure your attire doesn't restrict your exercises.

- **Yoga Mat:** A yoga mat provides a comfortable surface for floor exercises and helps prevent slipping.

- **Mirror:** Having a mirror in your exercise space can be beneficial for checking your posture and ensuring you're performing exercises correctly.

- **Props:** Depending on the exercises you choose, you might need props like resistance bands, yoga blocks, or a stability ball. These can add variety and challenge to your routine.

Safety Considerations Before we conclude this chapter, it's essential to touch on safety. Safety should always be a top priority when engaging in any exercise program, including pelvic floor exercises. Here are some safety considerations:

- **Consult a Healthcare Provider:** If you have any

medical conditions or concerns about your pelvic floor health, consult a healthcare provider or pelvic health specialist before starting an exercise routine.

- **Proper Form:** Pay close attention to your form during exercises. Using incorrect form can lead to injury or ineffectiveness.

- **Start Slowly:** If you're new to pelvic floor exercises, start slowly and gradually increase intensity. Pushing too hard too soon can lead to muscle strain.

- **Listen to Your Body:** If you experience pain or discomfort during exercises, stop immediately and reassess your technique. Pain is not a normal part of pelvic floor exercises.

In Summary Chapter 4 has provided essential guidance for preparing to embark on your pelvic floor exercise journey. By setting realistic goals, creating a comfortable exercise space, and identifying the necessary equipment and attire, you're setting yourself up for success. Remember, safety is paramount, so consult with a healthcare provider if you have any concerns about your pelvic floor health. As we progress through this book, we'll delve deeper into specific pelvic floor exercises and routines tailored to your goals and needs. So, get ready to strengthen and empower your pelvic floor in the upcoming chapters!

CHAPTER 5

Kegel Exercises

Welcome to Chapter 5, where we dive into the fundamentals of Kegel exercises. These exercises form the core of pelvic floor workouts and are a powerful tool for strengthening the pelvic floor muscles. In this chapter, we'll explore the basics of Kegels, various techniques and variations, and how to track your progress as you work toward a stronger and healthier pelvic floor.

Understanding the Basics of Kegel Exercises Kegel exercises, named after Dr. Arnold Kegel who developed them in the 1940s, are simple yet highly effective pelvic floor exercises. They target the pubococcygeus (PC) muscles, which are part of the pelvic floor. The primary goal of Kegels is to strengthen these muscles, enhancing their ability to support your pelvic organs and improve bladder and bowel control.

How to Do Kegel Exercises: The Basics Performing Kegels correctly is essential to reap their benefits. Here's a step-by-step guide to get you started:

1. **Find Your Pelvic Floor Muscles:** Begin by identifying the muscles you'll be working. Imagine you're trying to stop the flow of urine mid-stream or trying to prevent passing gas. The muscles you engage in these actions are your pelvic floor muscles.

2. **The "Squeeze" and "Lift":** Once you've located these muscles, contract and lift them. Avoid holding your breath or tightening your

buttocks, thighs, or abdomen. The contraction should focus solely on your pelvic floor.

3. **Hold and Release:** Squeeze and lift your pelvic floor muscles as strongly as you can without straining, and then hold this contraction for a few seconds (start with 3-5 seconds and gradually increase). After the hold, release and relax your muscles fully.

4. **Repeat:** Perform a set of repetitions. Start with 10-15 repetitions and gradually

increase as your muscles become stronger. Remember to rest between sets.

5. **Consistency is Key:** To see significant improvements, consistency is crucial. Aim to do Kegel exercises at least 3-4 times a week.

Variations and Techniques

Kegel exercises can be tailored to your specific needs and goals. Here are some variations and techniques to consider:

- **Quick Flicks:** These involve rapid contractions of the pelvic floor muscles.

Contract and release your pelvic floor muscles as quickly as possible, like a quick flick. Quick flicks are exccllent for enhancing muscle responsiveness.

- **Elevator Kegels:** Imagine your pelvic floor as an elevator with multiple floors. Contract your muscles gently, then increase the contraction intensity gradually, as if the elevator is moving up the floors. Then, release in the same gradual manner, as if the elevator is descending. This technique helps build both endurance and control.

- **Bridge Kegels:** Combine Kegels with a bridge exercise. Lie on your back with your knees bent and feet flat on the floor. As you lift your hips into a bridge position, contract your pelvic floor muscles. Hold for a few seconds, then lower your hips and release the contraction. This variation adds a strength-building component to your pelvic floor workout.

- **Balloon Blowing:** Pretend you're blowing up a balloon.

Inhale deeply and, as you exhale, contract your pelvic floor muscles as if you're blowing up the balloon. This technique synchronizes breath with pelvic floor contractions, promoting coordination and control.

Tracking Your Progress Like any exercise routine, it's important to track your progress to stay motivated and ensure you're on the right path. Here's how to monitor your journey:

- **Exercise Journal:** Maintain a journal to record your Kegel workouts. Note the number of repetitions, duration of holds, and any variations or techniques you're using. This journal will help you stay consistent and make adjustments as needed.

- **Strength and Control:** Pay attention to changes in your strength and control. Are you able to hold contractions longer? Can you contract more strongly? These improvements indicate progress.

- **Symptoms:** If you're practicing Kegels to address specific issues like urinary incontinence, track any changes in your symptoms. Are you experiencing fewer leaks? Is your bladder control improving? Document these changes to assess the effectiveness of your routine.

- **Consultation:** Consider scheduling regular check-ins with a pelvic health specialist or physical therapist. They can provide expert guidance, evaluate your progress, and suggest modifications to your routine.

In Summary Chapter 5 has provided a comprehensive overview of Kegel exercises, the cornerstone of pelvic floor workouts. You've learned how to perform Kegels correctly, explored variations and techniques, and discovered the importance of tracking your progress. With consistency and the right approach, Kegels can help you achieve a stronger, healthier pelvic floor, enhancing bladder and bowel control, supporting sexual health, and promoting overall well-being. In the upcoming chapters, we'll continue to expand your knowledge and skills, guiding you on your journey toward pelvic floor empowerment. So, let's keep moving forward, one Kegel at a time!

CHAPTER 6

Beyond Kegels: Comprehensive Pelvic Floor Workouts

Welcome to Chapter 6, where we go beyond the basics of Kegels to explore a comprehensive approach to pelvic floor exercises. While Kegels are a fundamental component, a well-rounded workout routine can provide even more benefits for your pelvic floor health. In this chapter, we'll delve into various approaches, including pelvic floor-focused yoga, Pilates for pelvic health, and combining cardio with pelvic floor exercises.

Pelvic Floor-Focused Yoga

Yoga is a versatile practice that can be adapted to focus specifically on pelvic floor health. Incorporating yoga into your pelvic floor workout routine can bring balance, flexibility, and relaxation to your muscles.

Poses for Pelvic Floor Health:

1. **Bridge Pose (Setu Bandha Sarvangasana):** This pose strengthens the pelvic floor muscles and

helps alleviate stress and tension.

2. **Child's Pose (Balasana):** Child's Pose can help relax and stretch the pelvic floor muscles, promoting flexibility.

3. **Cat-Cow Stretch:** The gentle arching and rounding of the spine in this sequence can help increase awareness of your pelvic floor muscles and promote circulation.

4. **Squat Pose (Malasana):** Squatting stretches and strengthens the pelvic floor muscles. You can modify this

pose based on your flexibility and comfort.

Breath Awareness: Yoga places a strong emphasis on breath control. Deep, diaphragmatic breathing can help relax and engage the pelvic floor muscles effectively. Combining breath awareness with pelvic floor-focused poses enhances your connection with these vital muscles.

Pilates for Pelvic Health

Pilates is another excellent choice for pelvic floor exercise. Pilates exercises focus on core strength, which includes the pelvic floor.

The controlled, precise movements of Pilates can help improve posture, alignment, and overall pelvic stability.

Pilates Exercises for Pelvic Floor Health:

1. **Pelvic Curl:** This exercise involves lifting your pelvis off the ground while engaging your core and pelvic floor muscles.
2. **Single Leg Stretch:** While performing this exercise, you engage your deep core muscles, including the pelvic floor, as you extend and bend your legs.

3. **The Hundred:** In this exercise, you maintain a curled position while pumping your arms. This engages your core, including the pelvic floor, for an extended period.

4. **Saw:** The Saw is a seated exercise that combines rotation and stretching while engaging the core and pelvic floor muscles.

Breath Coordination: Pilates emphasizes proper breathing techniques, which can be synchronized with pelvic floor muscle engagement. Learning to coordinate your breath with your movements is a fundamental aspect of Pilates and can enhance your pelvic floor workout.

Combining Cardio and Pelvic Floor Exercises Cardiovascular exercises like walking, swimming, or cycling can be integrated with pelvic floor exercises to create a well-rounded routine.

Cardiovascular Benefits: Cardio exercises promote overall health and can help with weight management. Maintaining a healthy weight reduces the strain on your pelvic floor, benefiting its function.

Interval Training: Incorporating short bursts of high-intensity exercises, such as jumping jacks or running in place, between sets of pelvic floor exercises can elevate your heart rate and add an element of cardio to your workout.

Precautions: It's essential to exercise caution when incorporating cardio, especially high-impact activities. If you're dealing with pelvic floor issues or have recently given birth, consult with a healthcare provider or pelvic health specialist to determine the most appropriate cardio exercises for your condition.

Sample Comprehensive Pelvic Floor Workout Routine:

1. **Warm-Up:** Start with 5-10 minutes of light cardio, such as brisk walking, to get your blood flowing and prepare your muscles for exercise.

2. **Pelvic Floor Exercises:** Perform a set of Kegels, focusing on proper form and control. Start with 10-15 repetitions, gradually increasing over time.

3. **Yoga or Pilates:** Choose 20-30 minutes of yoga or Pilates exercises focused on pelvic floor health. Follow instructional videos or attend classes if needed.

4. **Interval Cardio:** Incorporate 10-15 minutes of interval cardio exercises to elevate your heart rate. Ensure you're maintaining proper pelvic floor engagement during these exercises.

5. **Cool Down:** Finish your workout with 5-10 minutes of gentle stretching and relaxation exercises, such as

deep breathing or meditation.

In Summary Chapter 6 has introduced a comprehensive approach to pelvic floor exercises, moving beyond Kegels to incorporate yoga, Pilates, and cardio. These exercises offer a holistic way to strengthen and maintain your pelvic floor health, addressing not only muscle strength but also flexibility, posture, and cardiovascular fitness. As you continue your journey, remember that consistency is key. Combine various exercises to create a routine that suits your goals and needs, and always listen to your body. In the following chapters, we'll explore additional aspects of pelvic floor health, including nutrition, lifestyle factors, and exercises tailored for specific populations. So, keep up the great work, and let's continue working toward a stronger, healthier you!

CHAPTER 7

Nutrition and Pelvic Floor Health

Welcome to Chapter 7, where we'll explore the crucial connection between nutrition and pelvic floor health. Just as exercise plays a vital role in strengthening your pelvic floor, what you eat can significantly impact its function and overall well-being. In this chapter, we'll delve into the ways that your diet can influence your pelvic floor health, foods that support pelvic floor health, and the importance of hydration in this context.

The Impact of Diet on Pelvic Floor Health Your diet has a profound influence on your overall health, and your pelvic floor is no exception. What you eat can affect your weight, bowel regularity, hormonal balance, and even your muscles' ability to function correctly. Here's how your diet can impact your pelvic floor health:

1. **Weight Management:** Maintaining a healthy weight is crucial for pelvic floor health. Excess weight puts added pressure on your

pelvic organs and muscles, potentially weakening them and contributing to issues like urinary incontinence or pelvic organ prolapse.

2. **Constipation:** A diet lacking in fiber can lead to constipation, which can strain the pelvic floor muscles during bowel movements. Chronic straining can weaken these muscles over time.

3. **Hormonal Balance:** Hormones play a role in pelvic floor health, especially for women. A balanced diet can help regulate hormone

levels, particularly during menopause, which can impact pelvic floor function.

4. **Inflammation:** An inflammatory diet can contribute to general inflammation in the body, potentially affecting the pelvic floor muscles. Reducing inflammatory foods can help maintain pelvic health.

Foods That Support Pelvic Floor Health Now, let's explore the types of foods that can benefit your pelvic floor health:

1. **Fiber-Rich Foods:** A diet high in fiber promotes regular bowel movements, reducing the risk of constipation and straining. Include whole grains, fruits, vegetables, and legumes in your diet.

2. **Lean Proteins:** Protein is essential for muscle health, including the muscles of the pelvic floor. Opt for lean sources like poultry, fish, tofu, and beans.

3. **Healthy Fats:** Omega-3 fatty acids, found in fatty fish like salmon and flaxseeds, have anti-

inflammatory properties that can support overall pelvic health.

4. **Antioxidant-Rich Foods:** Antioxidants help reduce inflammation and support tissue health. Include a variety of colorful fruits and vegetables in your diet to get a broad spectrum of antioxidants.

5. **Probiotic Foods:** Probiotics promote gut health, which is linked to overall well-being, including pelvic floor health. Yogurt, kefir, sauerkraut, and kimchi

are good sources of probiotics.

6. **Hydrating Foods:** Staying hydrated is essential for preventing urinary tract infections (UTIs) and maintaining optimal bladder function. Include hydrating foods like watermelon, cucumber, and citrus fruits in your diet.

7. **Pelvic Health Superfoods:** Some foods are particularly beneficial for pelvic health. These include but are not limited to:

   - **Berries:** Rich in antioxidants and fiber,

berries help combat inflammation and support digestive health.

- **Leafy Greens:** Packed with vitamins, minerals, and fiber, leafy greens like spinach and kale promote overall well-being, including pelvic health.

- **Nuts and Seeds:** Almonds, walnuts, chia seeds, and flaxseeds provide healthy fats and fiber, which benefit the pelvic floor.

- **Ginger and Turmeric:** These spices have anti-inflammatory properties that can help alleviate pelvic pain and discomfort.

Hydration and Its Role in Pelvic Floor Health Staying adequately hydrated is a crucial aspect of pelvic floor health. Dehydration can lead to issues like urinary tract infections and constipation, which can place stress on the pelvic floor. Here's why hydration matters:

1. **Bladder Function:** A well-hydrated body ensures that your bladder can function optimally. Dehydration can lead to concentrated urine, which can irritate the bladder lining and increase the risk of UTIs.

2. **Digestive Health:** Proper hydration supports regular bowel movements, reducing the likelihood of constipation and straining during bowel movements. Straining can weaken the

pelvic floor muscles over time.

3. **Muscle Function:** Adequate fluid intake helps maintain muscle function, including the muscles of the pelvic floor. Dehydration can lead to muscle cramps and decreased muscle performance.

4. **Overall Well-Being:** Staying hydrated promotes overall well-being, which is essential for maintaining pelvic floor health. When you feel good, your body is better equipped to function optimally.

Practical Tips for Staying Hydrated:

1. **Listen to Your Body:** Pay attention to your body's thirst cues. Thirst is a signal that it's time to hydrate.

2. **Carry a Water Bottle:** Keep a reusable water bottle with you throughout the day. This serves as a visual reminder to drink water.

3. **Set Hydration Goals:** Establish daily hydration goals based on your individual needs. Aim for a specific number of glasses or ounces per day.

4. **Incorporate Hydrating Foods:** As mentioned earlier, foods like watermelon, cucumber, and citrus fruits have high water content and can contribute to your hydration.

5. **Avoid Excessive Caffeine and Alcohol:** Both caffeine and alcohol can have diuretic effects, increasing fluid loss. Consume them in moderation and balance with water intake.

In Summary Chapter 7 has shed light on the essential relationship between nutrition and pelvic floor health. Your diet plays a significant role in maintaining a healthy pelvic floor by supporting weight management, regular bowel movements, hormonal balance, and reducing inflammation. By incorporating foods that support pelvic health and staying adequately hydrated, you can promote the well-being of your pelvic floor and overall health. As we continue through this book, we'll explore additional factors that contribute to pelvic floor health, including lifestyle considerations and exercises tailored for specific populations. So, stay hydrated and keep nourishing your pelvic floor for a stronger, healthier you!

CHAPTER 8

Lifestyle and Pelvic Floor Health

Welcome to Chapter 8, where we'll delve into the impact of lifestyle on pelvic floor health. Beyond exercises and nutrition, how you live your daily life can have a substantial influence on the strength and function of your pelvic floor. In this chapter, we'll explore key lifestyle factors, such as posture, stress management, and habits related to toileting and lifting, that play a role in maintaining a healthy pelvic floor.

Posture and Pelvic Floor Health The way you carry yourself can significantly affect your pelvic floor. Proper posture is essential for providing optimal support to this area. Here's how posture impacts pelvic floor health:

1. **Sitting Posture:** When sitting for extended periods, maintain good posture. Sit with your feet flat on the floor and your back straight. Avoid crossing your legs,

which can put pressure on the pelvic floor.

2. **Standing Posture:** Stand tall with your weight evenly distributed on both feet. Engage your core muscles, including the pelvic floor, to support your spine.

3. **Lifting Posture:** Proper lifting techniques are vital for pelvic floor health. When lifting heavy objects, bend your knees, not your waist, and engage your core muscles, including the pelvic floor, to support the lift.

4. **Sleeping Posture:** Even your sleeping position can

impact your pelvic floor. Sleeping on your back with a pillow under your knees can help maintain proper alignment.

5. **Yoga and Pilates:** The practices of yoga and Pilates often emphasize posture, alignment, and core engagement. Regular participation in these activities can help improve your overall posture and benefit your pelvic floor.

Stress Management and Pelvic Floor Health Stress can manifest in various ways throughout the body, including the pelvic floor. Chronic stress can lead to muscle tension, poor posture, and altered breathing patterns, all of which can affect pelvic floor function. Here's how stress management is linked to pelvic floor health:

1. **Breathing Techniques:** Deep, diaphragmatic breathing can help relax the pelvic floor muscles and reduce tension. Incorporate mindfulness or meditation practices that focus on deep breathing to manage stress.

2. **Yoga and Relaxation:** Yoga and relaxation exercises can help release tension in the pelvic floor caused by stress. These practices promote mindfulness and body awareness, allowing you to identify and release areas of tension.

3. **Biofeedback Therapy:** Biofeedback therapy can assist in learning to control and relax the pelvic floor muscles. This therapy uses sensors to provide real-time feedback on muscle activity, helping you become more

aware of and manage muscle tension caused by stress.

4. **Stress Reduction Techniques:** Explore stress reduction techniques such as progressive muscle relaxation, guided imagery, or mindfulness meditation. These practices can help relax your entire body, including the pelvic floor.

Toileting Habits and Pelvic Floor Health Your toileting habits can have a significant impact on pelvic floor health, especially for women. Here are some habits to consider:

1. **Voiding Regularly:** Don't delay going to the restroom when you feel the urge to urinate. Holding in urine can weaken the pelvic floor muscles over time.

2. **Proper Wiping:** After using the restroom, be gentle when wiping, and avoid excessive wiping, as it can irritate the pelvic area.

3. **Constipation Management:** If you struggle with constipation, consider dietary changes, such as increasing fiber intake, to promote regular bowel movements. Avoid

straining during bowel movements, as this can strain the pelvic floor muscles.

4. **Pelvic Floor Relaxation:** When urinating, try to relax your pelvic floor muscles fully. Avoid straining or pushing to empty your bladder.

Lifting and Pelvic Floor Health Proper lifting techniques are crucial to protect your pelvic floor. Whether you're lifting heavy objects, groceries, or a child, here are some tips to keep in mind:

1. **Engage Your Core:** Before lifting, engage your core muscles, including the pelvic floor, to provide support to your spine and pelvis.

2. **Bend Your Knees:** When lifting heavy objects from the ground, bend your knees and keep your back straight. This technique reduces strain on your pelvic floor and lower back.

3. **Hold Objects Close:** Keep objects you're lifting close to your body to minimize strain on your back and pelvic floor muscles.

4. **Avoid Twisting:** When carrying something heavy, avoid twisting your torso. Instead, pivot your feet to change direction.

Sexual Health and Pelvic Floor Health Your sexual health is intimately connected to your pelvic floor. The pelvic floor muscles play a role in sexual function, including arousal, sensation, and orgasm. Here's how you can support your sexual health in relation to your pelvic floor:

1. **Pelvic Floor Exercises:** Regular pelvic floor exercises can enhance sexual function

by increasing blood flow and muscle tone in the pelvic region.

2. **Open Communication:** Maintain open and honest communication with your partner about your sexual health and any concerns related to pelvic floor function.

3. **Pelvic Pain:** If you experience pelvic pain during sexual activity, consult a healthcare provider or pelvic health specialist for evaluation and treatment options.

4. **Kegels and Sensation:** Some individuals may find that practicing Kegel exercises increases sexual sensation and pleasure. Experiment with different techniques to discover what works best for you.

In Summary Chapter 8 has emphasized the importance of lifestyle factors in maintaining pelvic floor health. Proper posture, stress management, toileting habits, and lifting techniques all contribute to the well-being of your pelvic floor. By incorporating mindful practices and habits into your daily life, you can support and strengthen your pelvic floor, promoting overall health and well-being. As we continue through this book, we'll explore exercises tailored to specific populations and provide guidance for lifelong pelvic floor health. So, keep making these positive lifestyle changes and prioritize your pelvic floor health for a stronger, healthier you!

CHAPTER 9

Pelvic Floor Health Across the Lifespan

Welcome to Chapter 9, where we'll discuss how pelvic floor health varies across the different stages of life. Just as our bodies change over time, so do the needs and challenges of our pelvic floor muscles. In this chapter, we'll explore pelvic floor health from childhood to old age, addressing the unique considerations, exercises, and preventive measures for each stage.

Childhood and Adolescence: Laying the Foundation The journey of pelvic floor health begins in childhood and adolescence. While these young years may not seem relevant to pelvic floor health, they lay the foundation for a healthy pelvic floor in the future.

Considerations:

1. **Education:** It's essential to educate children and adolescents about their pelvic floor and its importance. Teach them about healthy toileting habits, the role of the pelvic

floor in bladder and bowel control, and the significance of hydration.

2. **Physical Activity:** Encourage regular physical activity to promote overall muscle tone and health, including the pelvic floor muscles.

3. **Hydration:** Teach children the importance of staying hydrated to maintain a healthy bladder and bowel function.

Exercises:

1. **Healthy Habits:** Focus on developing habits like

regular exercise and good posture from a young age. These habits support pelvic floor health throughout life.

2. **Kegel Awareness:** While Kegel exercises may not be necessary during childhood and adolescence, awareness of pelvic floor muscles can be introduced. Simple cues like "squeeze and lift" can help children become conscious of these muscles.

Young Adulthood: Reproductive and Lifestyle Changes In young adulthood, reproductive health and lifestyle choices can significantly impact the pelvic floor.

Considerations:

1. **Pregnancy and Childbirth:** For women, pregnancy and childbirth can place stress on the pelvic floor. Prenatal education and postpartum recovery exercises are essential.

2. **Weight Management:** Maintaining a healthy weight is crucial to reduce the strain on the pelvic floor.

3. **High-Impact Exercise:** Engaging in high-impact exercises without proper

pelvic floor support can lead to issues like urinary incontinence. Learning to engage the pelvic floor during exercise is vital.

4. **Sexual Health:** Open communication about sexual health and any discomfort during intercourse is essential.

Exercises:

1. **Pelvic Floor Exercises During Pregnancy:** Prenatal exercises can help prepare the pelvic floor for childbirth. Consult a healthcare provider or pelvic

health specialist for guidance on safe exercises.

2. **Postpartum Recovery:** After childbirth, postpartum exercises can assist in healing and strengthening the pelvic floor.

3. **Pelvic Floor Awareness:** Promote awareness of pelvic floor health and the benefits of Kegel exercises. Young adults can start incorporating regular Kegel routines into their fitness regimens.

Middle Adulthood: Changes in Hormones and Lifestyle As

people move into middle adulthood, hormonal changes and lifestyle factors continue to influence pelvic floor health.

Considerations:

1. **Hormonal Changes:** Menopause brings hormonal shifts that can affect the pelvic floor. These changes may lead to vaginal dryness, discomfort, or changes in sexual function.

2. **Weight Management:** Maintaining a healthy weight remains essential for pelvic floor health.

3. **Lifestyle Factors:** Stress, high-impact exercise, and dietary choices can impact the pelvic floor.

Exercises:

1. **Kegels for Menopause:** Kegel exercises can help alleviate some menopausal symptoms, such as urinary incontinence and vaginal discomfort.

2. **Core Strengthening:** Incorporate exercises that strengthen the core, as a strong core supports the pelvic floor.

Late Adulthood: Aging and Maintaining Pelvic Health In late adulthood, aging plays a significant role in pelvic floor health. Maintaining a strong pelvic floor becomes even more critical.

Considerations:

1. **Pelvic Organ Prolapse:** Aging increases the risk of pelvic organ prolapse. Awareness and preventive measures are essential.

2. **Osteoporosis:** Osteoporosis can affect the pelvic bones, potentially impacting the pelvic floor. Weight-bearing exercises

and dietary calcium intake are vital.

3. **Bladder and Bowel Changes:** Age-related changes in bladder and bowel function may occur. Adequate hydration, fiber intake, and pelvic floor exercises can help manage these changes.

Exercises:

1. **Pelvic Floor Maintenance:** Continue with regular pelvic floor exercises to maintain muscle strength and function.

2. **Balance and Flexibility:** Incorporate exercises that promote balance and flexibility to prevent falls and injuries that could impact the pelvic floor.

In Summary Chapter 9 has explored pelvic floor health across the lifespan, addressing the unique considerations and exercises for each stage of life. From childhood to late adulthood, maintaining a healthy pelvic floor requires awareness, education, and consistent exercises tailored to your specific needs. By proactively addressing pelvic floor health throughout life, you can promote overall well-being and enjoy the benefits of a strong and resilient pelvic floor. In the final chapter, we'll bring together all the knowledge and strategies discussed in this book to create a holistic approach to pelvic floor health that you can integrate into your life for a lifetime of well-being. So, let's continue on this journey toward a stronger, healthier pelvic floor!

CHAPTER 10

A Lifetime of Pelvic Floor Health

Welcome to the final chapter of our journey towards pelvic floor health. In this chapter, we'll bring together all the knowledge, strategies, and exercises discussed throughout this book to create a comprehensive, lifelong approach to pelvic floor health. Whether you're starting your journey or have been on it for some time, these guidelines will help you maintain a strong and healthy pelvic floor throughout your life.

The Lifelong Approach

Maintaining pelvic floor health is not a one-time endeavor; it's a lifelong commitment. Just as you care for your overall health through diet, exercise, and regular check-ups, your pelvic floor deserves the same attention. Here's how you can integrate pelvic floor care into your life:

1. Awareness and Education

- **Know Your Pelvic Floor:** Understanding the anatomy and function of your pelvic floor is the first step. Knowledge empowers you to make informed decisions about your health.

- **Stay Informed:** Keep up with developments in pelvic health. New exercises, techniques, and therapies continually emerge.

2.   Consistent   Exercise Routine

- **Kegel Exercises:** Continue incorporating Kegel exercises into your routine. These exercises are the foundation of pelvic floor health and can be adapted to your changing needs.

- **Variety is Key:** As you progress, include a variety of pelvic floor exercises to challenge and strengthen your muscles further. Yoga, Pilates, and core workouts are excellent options.

- **Regularity:** Consistency is key. Aim to perform pelvic floor exercises at least three to four times a week.

3. Proper Nutrition and Hydration

- **Balanced Diet:** Maintain a balanced diet rich in fiber, lean proteins, healthy fats, and antioxidant-rich foods. These choices support overall health and aid in pelvic floor function.

- **Stay Hydrated:** Hydration is vital for bladder and bowel health. Aim for adequate daily water intake, and incorporate hydrating foods into your diet.

4. Lifestyle Considerations

- **Posture Awareness:** Maintain good posture, whether sitting, standing, or lifting. Proper alignment supports your pelvic floor muscles.

- **Stress Management:** Incorporate stress-reduction techniques into your daily life, such as meditation, mindfulness, or relaxation exercises. Chronic stress can strain the pelvic floor.

- **Toileting Habits:** Continue healthy toileting habits, including voiding regularly and avoiding straining during bowel movements.

- **Weight Management:** Maintain a healthy weight to

reduce excess pressure on the pelvic floor.

5. Sexual Health

- **Open Communication:** Maintain open communication with your partner about your sexual health and any changes or concerns related to pelvic floor function.
- **Consult a Specialist:** If you experience sexual discomfort or pain related to your pelvic floor, consult a healthcare provider or pelvic health specialist for

evaluation and treatment
options.

6. Pregnancy and Postpartum Care

- **Prenatal Exercises:** If you become pregnant, consider prenatal exercises to prepare your pelvic floor for childbirth.
- **Postpartum Recovery:** After childbirth, engage in postpartum exercises to aid in healing and strengthening the pelvic floor.

7. Aging Gracefully

- **Regular Pelvic Floor Maintenance:** Continue regular pelvic floor exercises, even as you age, to maintain muscle strength and function.

- **Osteoporosis Awareness:** Stay informed about osteoporosis and include weight-bearing exercises and sufficient calcium intake in your routine.

8. Healthcare Check-ups

- **Pelvic Health Specialist:** Schedule regular check-ups with a pelvic health specialist or physical therapist, especially if you have specific concerns or conditions related to your pelvic floor.

- **Annual Check-ups:** Include pelvic floor health discussions in your annual health check-ups with your primary care provider or gynecologist.

Creating Your Personalized Plan

Your lifelong approach to pelvic floor health should be personalized to your unique needs and circumstances. Here's how to create a plan tailored to you:

1. Assess Your Current Health

- **Consider Your Age:** Take into account your current stage of life and any specific needs or challenges you may face.

- **Evaluate Your Habits:** Reflect on your current diet, exercise routine, posture, stress management techniques, and toileting habits.

2. Set Clear Goals

- **Identify Objectives:** Determine your primary objectives. Are you looking to prevent issues, manage symptoms, or enhance pelvic health for a specific reason, such as pregnancy or athletic performance?

- **Realistic Goals:** Set achievable goals that you can track and adjust over time.

3. Create Your Plan

- **Exercise Routine:** Develop a well-rounded exercise routine that includes pelvic floor exercises, core workouts, and flexibility and balance exercises.

- **Diet and Hydration:** Adjust your diet to align with your goals for overall health and pelvic floor function.

- **Stress Management:** Implement stress-reduction techniques that resonate with you and fit into your daily life.

- **Lifestyle Factors:** Continuously evaluate your posture, toileting habits, and any lifestyle factors that may affect your pelvic floor.

4. Seek Professional Guidance

- **Consult a Specialist:** If you have specific concerns or conditions related to your pelvic floor, consult a pelvic health specialist or physical therapist for expert guidance.

- **Regular Check-ups:** Schedule regular check-ups with healthcare providers to monitor your overall health, including your pelvic floor.

5. Track Your Progress

- **Keep a Journal:** Maintain a journal to track your exercise routine, dietary changes, and any symptoms or improvements related to your pelvic floor.

- **Adjust as Needed:** Be flexible and willing to adjust your plan based on your progress and changing needs.

In Summary

Chapter 10 has outlined a comprehensive, lifelong approach to pelvic floor health. By integrating awareness, education, consistent exercises, proper nutrition, and lifestyle considerations into your daily life, you can maintain a strong and healthy pelvic floor at any age. Remember that your journey towards pelvic floor health is unique, and it should be adapted to your individual needs and circumstances. Regular check-ups with healthcare providers and specialists are essential to monitor your progress and address any concerns promptly. So, embrace this holistic approach, prioritize your pelvic floor health, and enjoy a lifetime of well-being and vitality!

CONCLUSION

In conclusion, this book has taken you on a transformative journey into the world of pelvic floor health. We've explored the intricate anatomy of the pelvic floor, delved into exercises that strengthen and support it, examined the profound influence of nutrition and lifestyle, and discussed the unique considerations for every stage of life. Through these chapters, we've strived to empower you with knowledge, practical tips, and a comprehensive approach to maintaining a strong and resilient pelvic floor.

Your pelvic floor health is not an isolated aspect of your well-being; it's an integral part of your overall health and vitality. Just as you care for your heart, muscles, and mind, your pelvic floor deserves attention and care throughout your life. By following the principles outlined in this book, you can:

1. **Prevent Issues:** Armed with knowledge and proactive measures, you can reduce the risk of pelvic floor disorders and complications.

2. **Manage Symptoms:** If
you're already experiencing
pelvic floor-related
symptoms, the exercises,
nutrition tips, and lifestyle
adjustments provided here
can help you manage and
improve your condition.

3. **Enhance Quality of Life:**
Whether you're a young
adult, in the prime of life, or
gracefully aging, a strong
pelvic floor contributes to
your overall well-being,
allowing you to enjoy life to
the fullest.

4. **Empower Yourself:**
Understanding your body

and its intricacies is a powerful form of self-care. It enables you to take control of your health and make informed decisions.

Remember that your pelvic floor journey is a lifelong one, and it's never too late to start. Regardless of your age, gender, or current pelvic health status, there is always room for improvement and maintenance. The principles presented in this book are adaptable to your unique circumstances, and they can be integrated seamlessly into your daily life.

Lastly, your pelvic floor health should never be a taboo topic. Share your knowledge with loved ones, start conversations, and encourage open dialogue about this vital aspect of health. By breaking down stigmas and sharing information, we can collectively work towards a world where everyone understands the importance of pelvic floor health and has the tools to maintain it.

Thank you for embarking on this journey with us. May your pelvic floor health journey be filled with strength, resilience, and a lifelong commitment to well-being. Here's to a healthier, happier you!